Single Surgical Procedures 26

A Colour Atlas of

Anterior Cervical Spine Fusion

Sean P.F. Hughes
MS, FRCSEd(ORTH), FRCSI, FRCS
*Professor, Department of Orthopaedic Surgery,
University of Edinburgh, Scotland.*

General Editor, Wolfe Surgical Atlases:
William F. Walker, DSc, ChM, FRCS (Edin. and England), FRS (Edin.).

Wolfe Medical Publications Ltd

General Editor, Wolfe Surgical Atlases:
William F. Walker, DSc, ChM, FRCS (Edin. and England), FRS (Edin.).

Copyright © Sean P.F. Hughes, 1985
Published by Wolfe Medical Publications Ltd, 1985
Printed by Royal Smeets Offset b.v.,
Weert, Netherlands
ISBN 0 7234 1042 9
ISSN 0264-8695

This book is one of the titles in the series of Wolfe Single Surgical Procedures, a series which will eventually cover some 200 titles.

If you wish to be kept informed of new additions to the series and receive details of our other titles, please write to Wolfe Medical Publications Ltd, Wolfe House, 3 Conway Street, London W1P 6HE.

All rights reserved. The contents of this book, both photographic and textual, may not be reproduced in any form, by print, photoprint, phototransparency, microfilm, microfiche, or any other means, nor may it be included in any computer retrieval system, without written permission from the publisher.

We list below a few of the other titles in print and in preparation in the Single Surgical Procedures series. Titles already published are marked (★); those titles to be published during the coming months are marked (●).

★*Parotidectomy*
★*Traditional Meniscectomy*
★*Inguinal Hernias & Hydroceles in Infants and Children*
★*Surgery for Pancreatic & Associated Carcinomata*
★*Subtotal Thyroidectomy*
★*Anterior Resection of Rectum*
★*Boari Bladder-Flap Procedure*
★*Surgery for Varicose Veins*
★*Treatment of Carpal Tunnel Syndrome*
★*Seromyotomy for Chronic Duodenal Ulcer*
★*Surgery for Undescended Testes*
★*Operations on the Internal Carotid Artery*
★*Renal Transplant*
★*Lumbar Discography*
★*Visceral Artery Reconstruction*
★*Minor Operations on the Hand*
★*Flexor Tendon Repair*
★*Proctocolectomy*
★*Common Operations of the Foot*
★*Right Hemicolectomy*
★*Extra-cranial and Intra-cranial Anastomosis*
★*Surgery for Hirschsprung's Disease*
★*Thyroid Lobectomy*
★*Surgery at the Thoracic Outlet*
●*Liver Transplantation*
●*Modified Radical Mastectomy*
●*Paratopic Transplant of Body and Tail of the Pancreas*
●*Subdiaphragmatic Total Gastrectomy for Malignant Disease*
●*Left Hemicolectomy*
Resection of Aortic Aneurysm
Ileorectal Anastomosis
Techniques of Nerve Grafting and Repair
Surgery for Dupuytren's Contracture
Athrodesis of the Ankle
Surgery for Congenital Dislocation of the Hip
Femoral and Tibial Osteotomy
Maxillo-Facial Traumatology
Surgery for Chondromalacia Patellae
Stabilisation for Extensive Spinal Injury
Spondylolisthesis
Laminectomy
Gall Bladder Cholecystectomy
Repair of Prolapsed Rectum
Resection of Oesophagus
Splenectomy
Anterior Nephrectomy
Bladder Augmentation
Caecocystoplasty
Hiatus Hernia
Total Gastrectomy
Billroth 1 Gastrectomy
Billroth 2 Gastrectomy
Abdominal Incisions
Thoracotomy
Chronic Pancreatitis Operation
Surgery for Strictures in Common Bile Duct
Biliary Enteric Anastomosis
Partial Hepatectomy
Splenectomy
Right Hemicolectomy
Appendicectomy
Incisional Hernia
Lung Lobectomy
Lung Removal
Gastric Reconstruction
Surgery for Lymphoedema
Dialysis Techniques
Surgery for Thoracic Outlet
Haemorrhoids
Abdominoperineal Resection of Rectum
Rectosigmoid Resection
Non-resectional Surgery for Multiple Bowel Stenosis
Surgery for Anorectal Incontinence
Craniotomy
Parathyroidectomy
Arterial Injuries
Arterial Bypass Grafts in Leg
Visceral Vascular Occlusion
Varicose Veins Surgery under Local Anaesthesia
Aortofemoral Bypass
Aortoiliac Disobliteration
Technique of Small Vessel Repair

Contents

Acknowledgements — 5

Introduction — 6

Clinical assessment and investigation — 7

Preparation for surgery — 15

Approach to cervical spine — 29

Instruments for curetting — 37

Disc removal — 39

Iliac crest exposed for graft — 46

Inserting the graft — 50

Sutures and dressings — 53

Postoperative observations — 56

Conclusion — 61

References — 62

Index — 63

Acknowledgements

I wish to express my most grateful thanks to Mr George Braddock, FRCS, Consultant Orthopaedic Surgeon, Ealing Hospital, who introduced me to this technique.

I also wish to thank Professor R. M. H. McMinn, Mr R. T. Hutchings, and Mr B. M. Logan for permitting me to use Figures 16 to 22 which have been taken from their book, *A Colour Atlas of Head and Neck Anatomy,* which is published by Wolfe Medical Publications.

I am also indebted to Mr Michael Devlin of the Photographic Department of Princess Margaret Rose Orthopaedic Hospital and Mrs Alison Rankin for typing the manuscript.

Introduction

The anterior approach to the cervical spine can be used for patients who have had:

a) Fracture dislocations of the cervical spine;
b) Tumours;
c) Infection;
d) Degenerative conditions.

Cervical spondylosis is the degenerative condition which lends itself to the anterior approach.
   Cervical spondylosis occurs usually in the older age groups and it is caused by disc degeneration or mechanical compression on the nerve root or spinal cord. Characteristically, patients present with pain in the base of the neck which radiates to the shoulder or to the skull. There may be significant limitation of the range of movements, probably flexion, extension and rotation; there may be also associated neurological signs of nerve root entrapment depending on which level is involved.

Clinical assessment and investigation

1 This patient presented with pain and difficulty in moving the neck for six months, which was due to cervical spondylosis. His head is held to one side. He complained of pain radiating into his left arm and shoulder. On examination he had motor weakness and sensory loss involving C6 and C7 nerve roots.

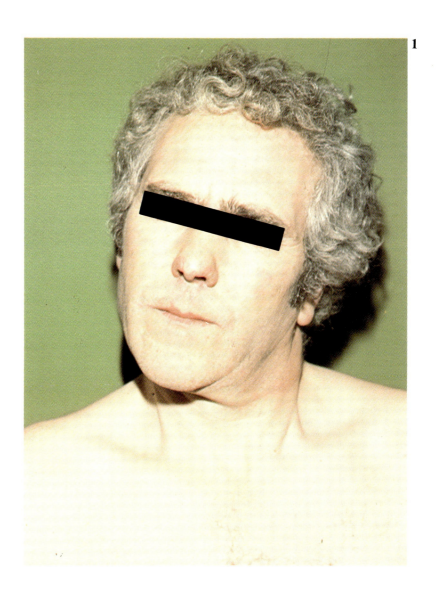

2 After the clinical examination the neck is xrayed to assess the degree of disc space narrowing that has occurred.

Disc degeneration may be apparent at several levels on the radiograph. However, the level that is the cause of the pain, is not necessarily the one with the most obvious disc space narrowing.

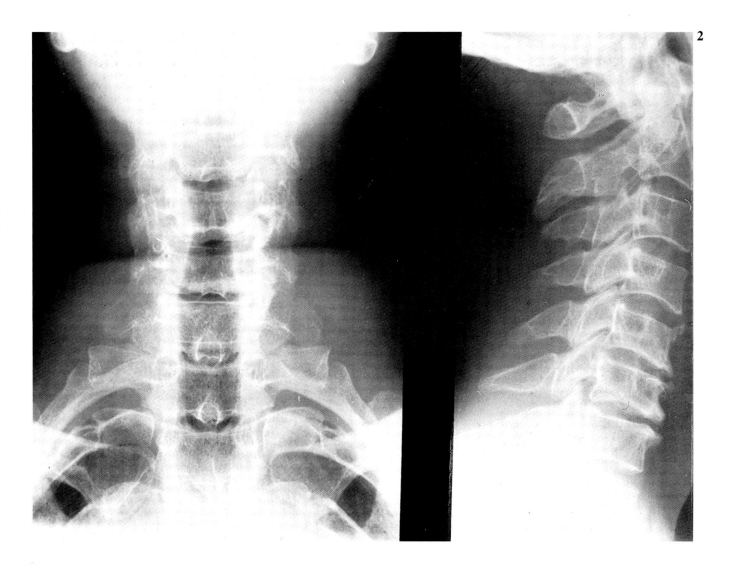

3 On the whole, oblique views are not that useful in detecting the disc that is the current cause of symptoms. The oblique views show narrowing and obliteration of the disc space and the nerve foramena. Also, they do not give any real indication of the degree of instability that may be occurring.

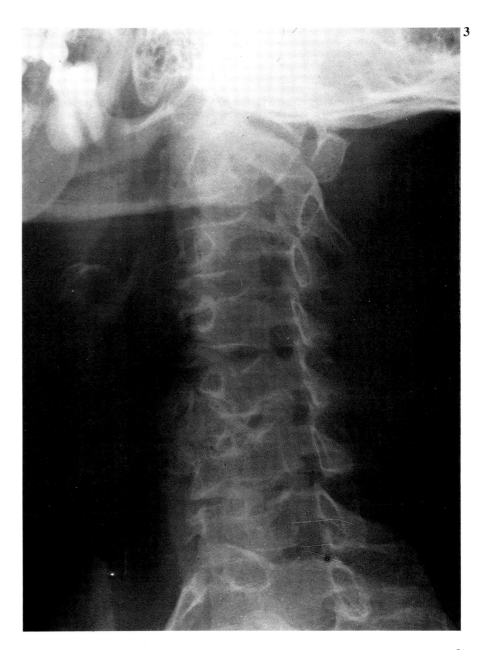

4 On the other hand flexion and extension views of the cervical spine are helpful, demonstrating where movement is occurring in the cervical column. The use of video to record cervical spine movement is also useful, to assess where movement occurs.

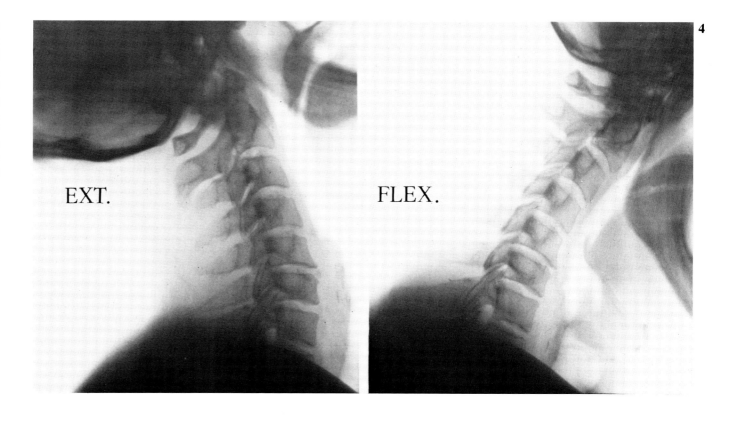

5 Contrast radiography helps to delineate the degree of nerve root compression. In this figure the contrast outlines the cervical cord and nerve roots and reveals compression at C5–6 levels in particular.

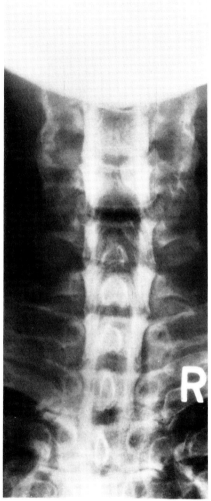

6 A barium swallow may help to demonstrate osteophyte formation. This radiograph shows the barium to be indented due to the new bone that has formed.

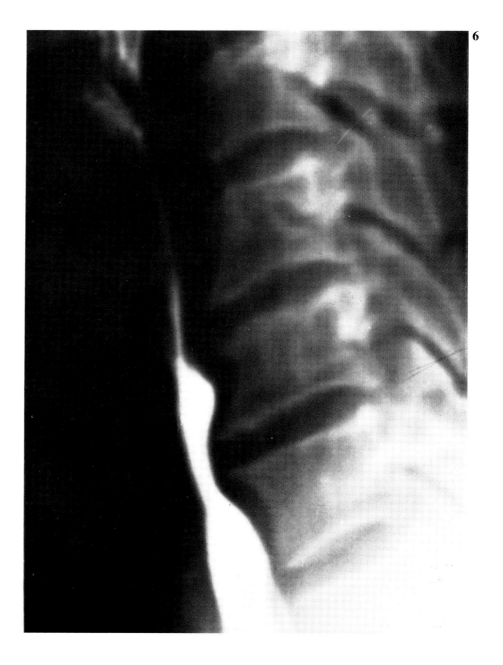

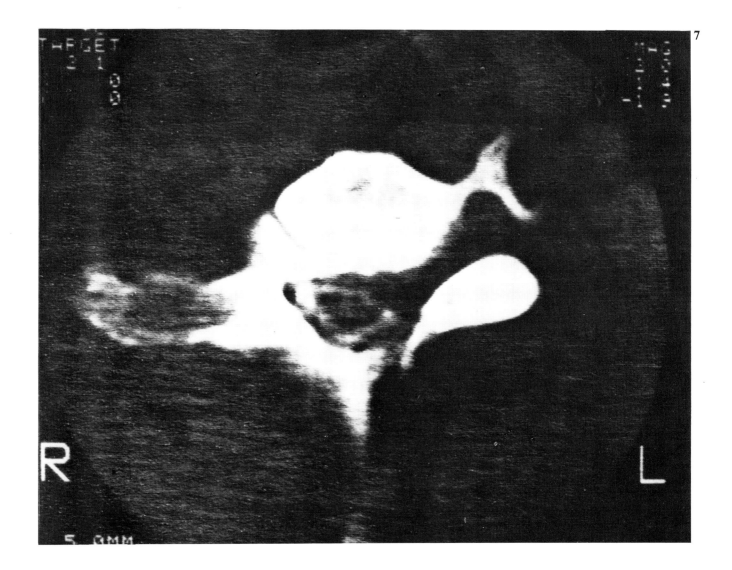

7 A computerised axial tomogram scan with a contrast medium can be used to demonstrate a filling defect pressing against the cord.
In this CAT scan there is compression of the cord.

8 A lateral view of the myelogram will demonstrate a herniation of the disc or if there is compression on the cord itself.

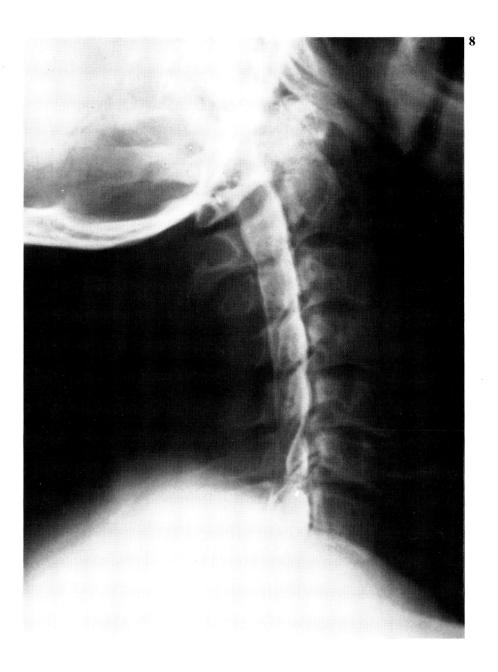

Preparation for surgery

After deciding to perform an anterior cervical decompression and fusion, based upon the clinical assessment and investigation, the following steps are taken using the technique described by Smith and Robinson (1958).

9 The patient is placed on the operating table with the neck in extension. It is important to place the neck in this position to gain access to the cervical spine. A sandbag may be placed under the shoulder.

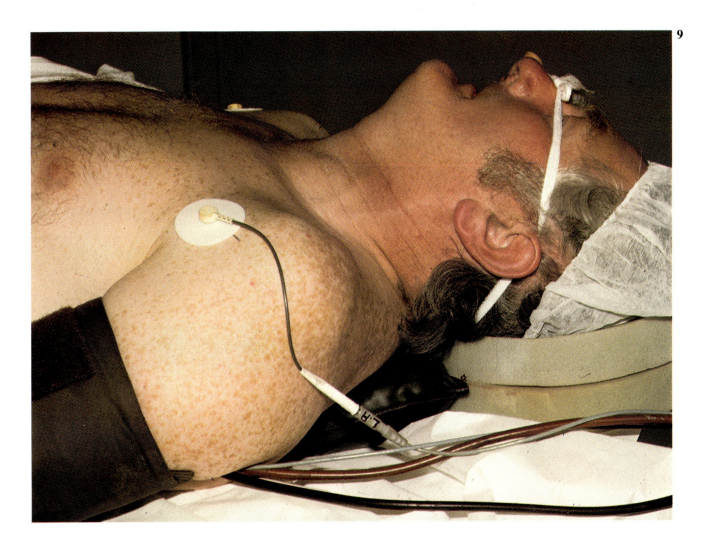

10 A halter is placed under the chin to allow distraction, before insertion of the graft. This halter is constructed easily and allows a longitudinal pull to be applied to the cervical column.

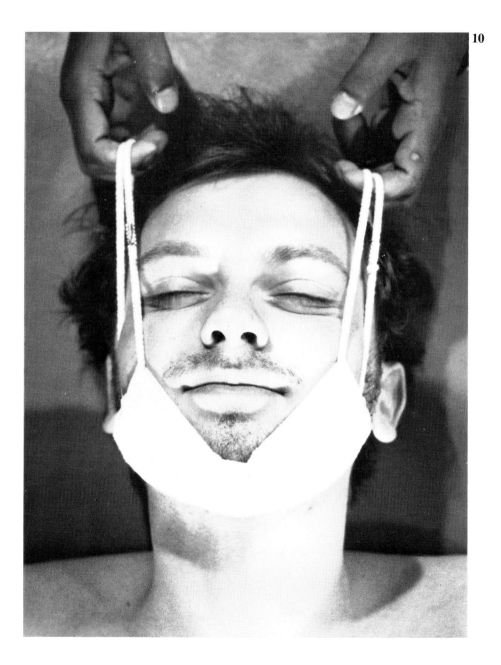

11 The patient is intubated and is positioned on the operating table in a slightly flexed angle, to allow easy direct visualisation of the neck and its structures. It is also important that the neck is held stable so that it does not lie to one side, as this can lead to difficulty in finding the correct approach through the neck.

Stability is best achieved by placing the head on a rubber ring and then putting small sandbags on either side of the head.

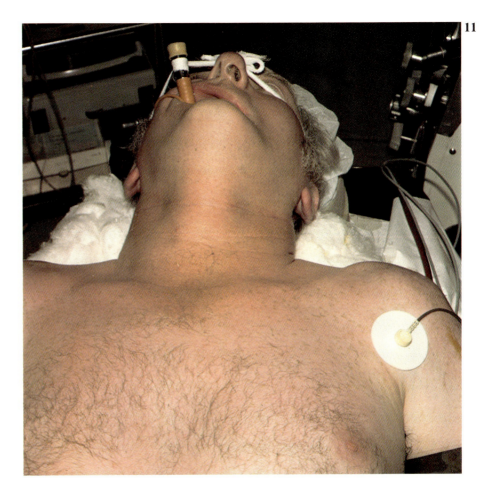

12 In side view the patient's head is stabilised and he is intubated, thus providing a clear view of the neck.

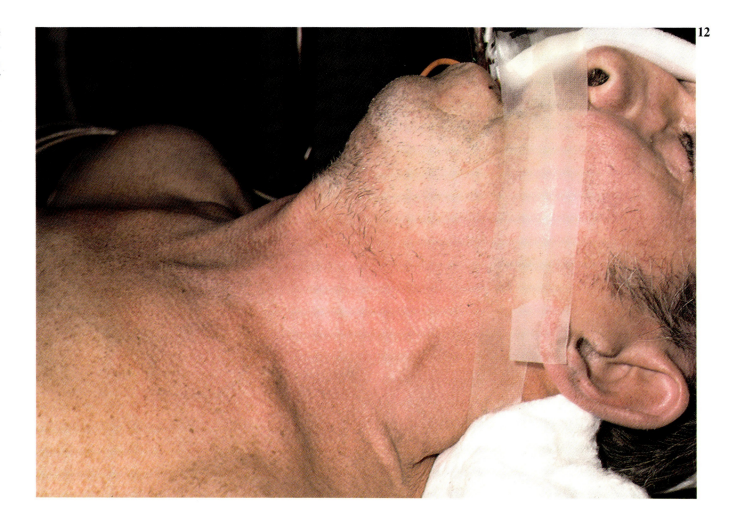

13 The patient is then draped and the donor site from the iliac crest area is also left exposed.

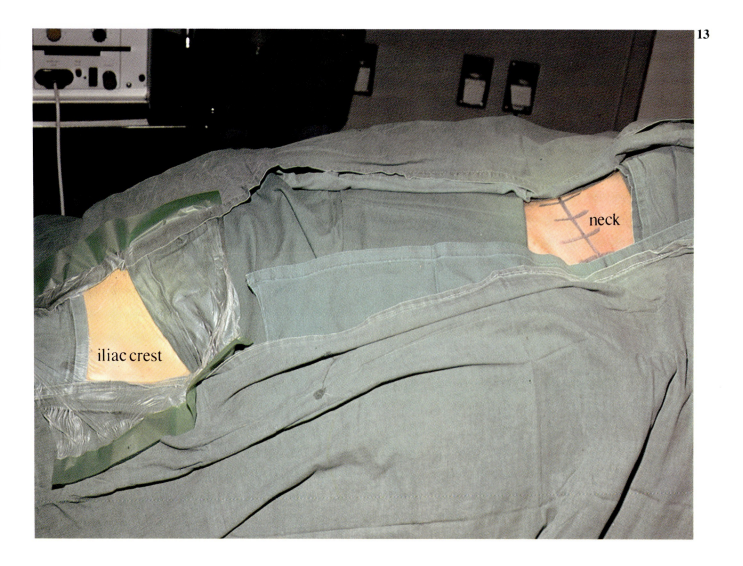

14 It is imperative that two assistants are present to retract the structures in the neck and to allow adequate exposure of the cervical spine. This is a most important step, for if only one assistant is available, it is extremely difficult to obtain a clear picture of the deep structures of the neck.

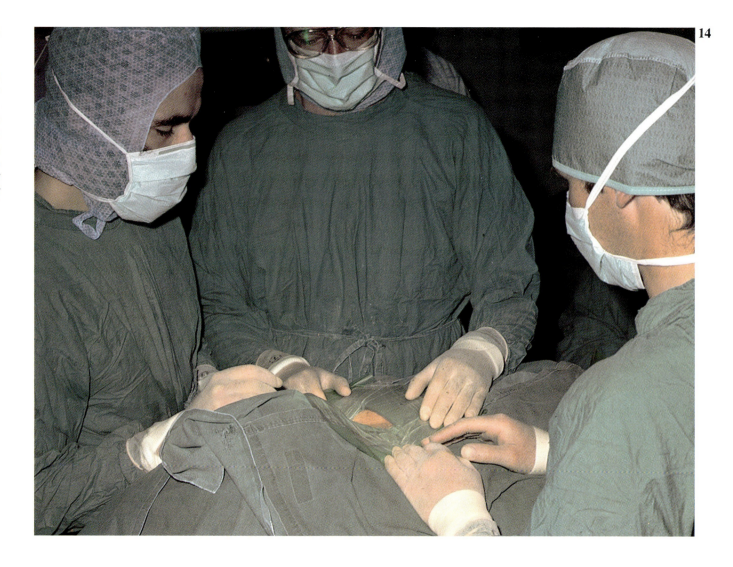

15 The bones of the cervical spine which can be approached. They are the seven cervical vertebrae, although it is impossible to reach C_1 from this approach, it is possible with careful dissection to reach from the lower border of C_2 down to T_1.

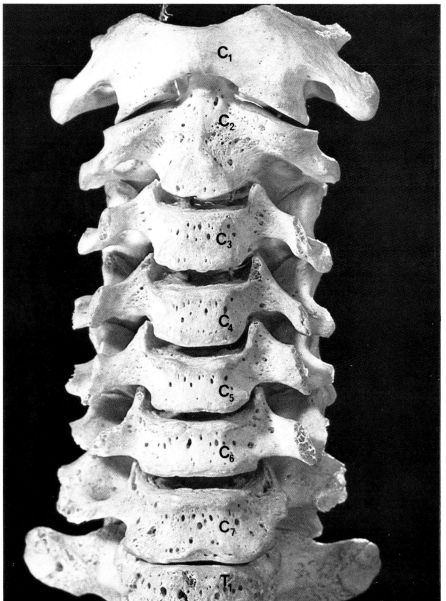

16 The surface markings of the neck demonstrating the anterior triangle of the neck and the following structures are defined:
1. Sternomastoid
2. Mandible
3. Thyroid cartilage
4. Carotid artery

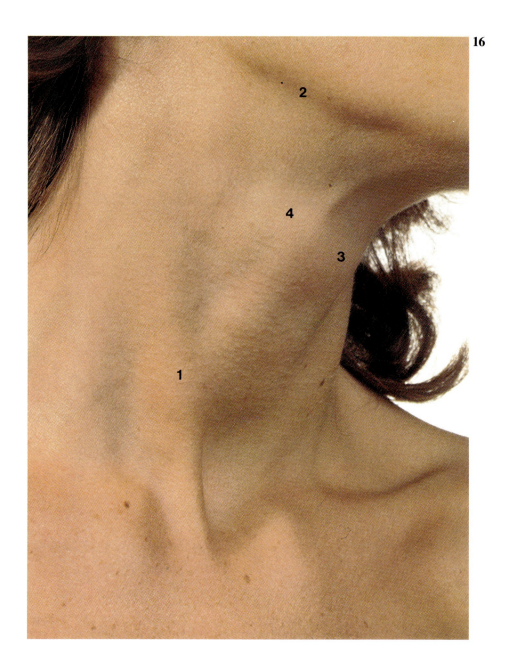

17 The neck. Superficial dissection I. The platysma is demonstrated.

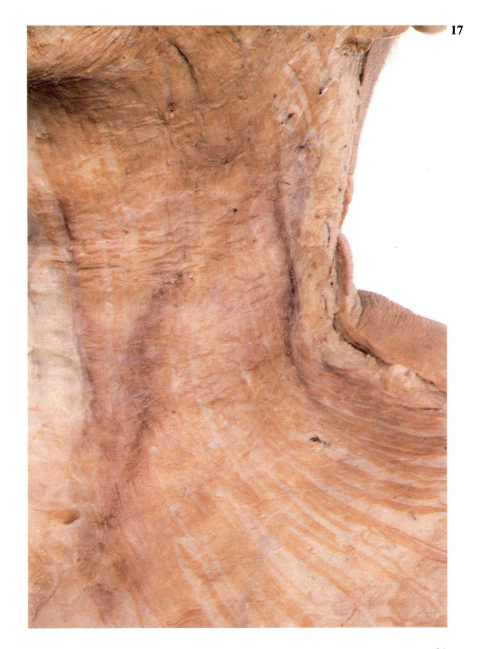

18 The neck. Superficial dissection, showing the anterior triangle of the neck on the left side, which is the area to approach the cervical column.
1 Sternomastoid
2 Anterior jugular vein

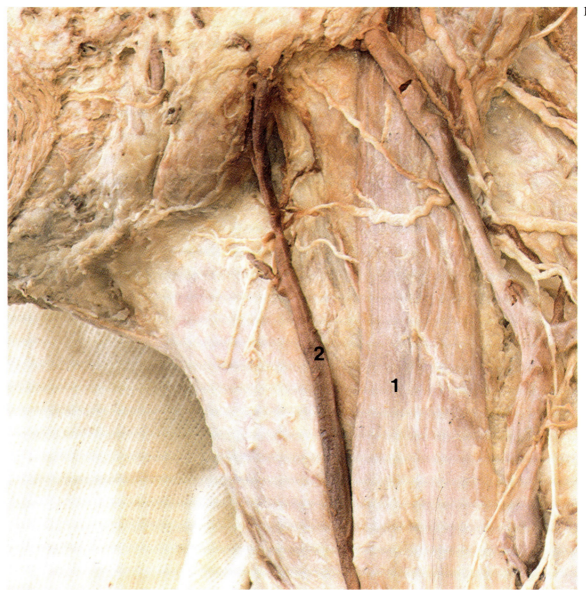

19 The neck. Superficial dissection. This shows the anterior triangle of the neck on the left, demonstrating the relationship of the vessels coming from the external carotid.
1 Common carotid artery
2 External carotid artery
3 Sternomastoid
4 Sternohoid
5 Omohyoid

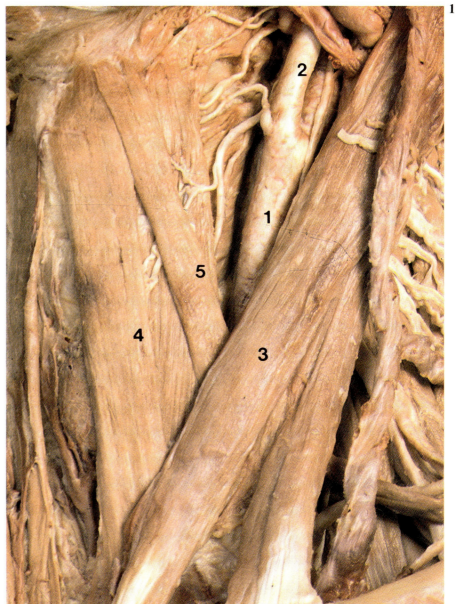

20 Deep dissection of the neck showing the thyroid gland, the middle thyroid vein and the common carotid artery and jugular vein. The plane to be developed is between the common carotid artery and the thyroid in the trachea, with the oesophagus deep to this.
   1 Common carotid artery
   2 Internal jugular vein
   3 Thyroid gland
   4 Middle thyroid vein
   5 Inferior thyroid artery
   6 Inferior thyroid vein

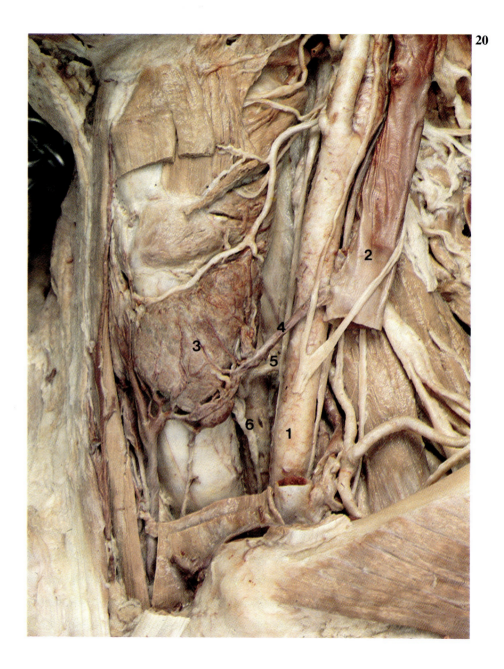

21 Deep dissection. In this dissection, the cervical vertebrae have been exposed and the muscles on the front of the neck demonstrated.
 1 Oesophagus and trachea
 2 Cervical column
 3 Longus colii muscle

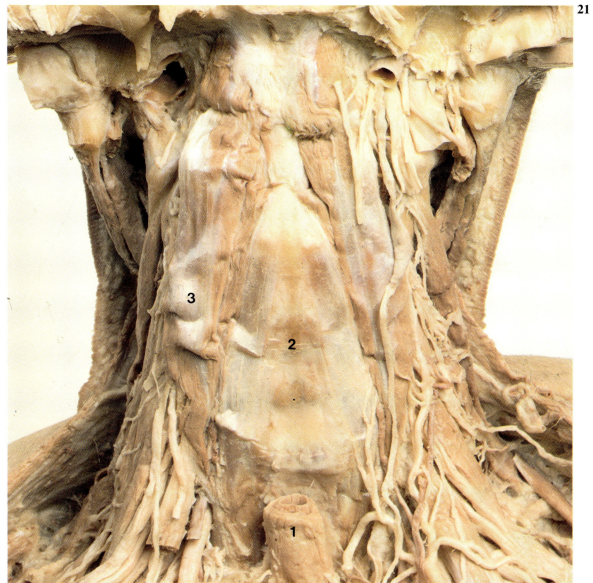

22 The right half of a sagittal section of the lower part of the head and neck, slightly to the left of the midline. The relationships between the oesophagus and the cervical column can be seen.
   1 Trachea
   2 Oesophagus
   3 Vertebra C3
   4 Disc
   5 Spinal cord

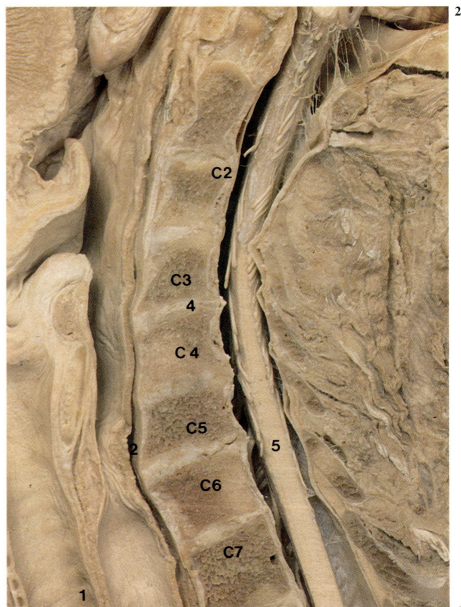

The approach to the cervical spine

23 An oblique incision is made through the skin on the left hand side. The neck can equally well be approached from the right hand side. The left hand side is chosen in this patient. C3 to C7 can be reached relatively easily through this approach. **However, it is important to remember the thoracic duct is on the left side at the T1 level.**

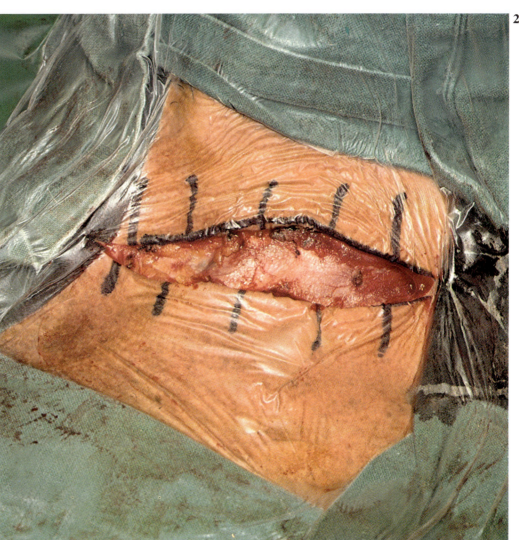

24 The platysma muscle is divided in the line of the incision, care being taken of the anterior jugular vein. The sternomastoid muscle is not necessarily divided, in order to gain exposure, and can be left intact, and retracted laterally.

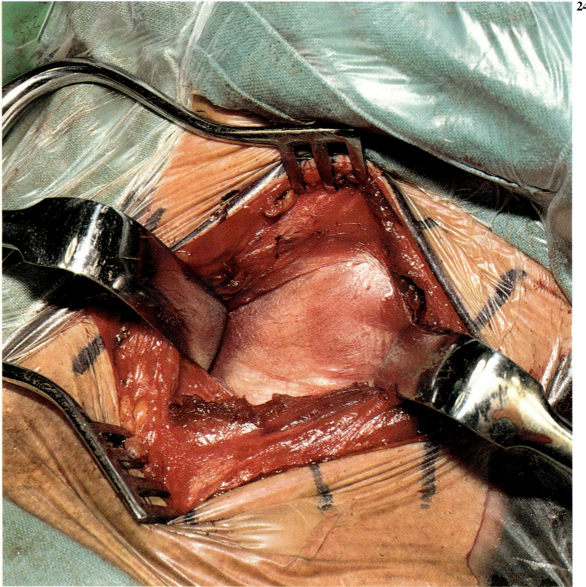

25 The plane lying between the trachea and oesophagus medially and the carotid artery and the jugular vein laterally, is identified. **It is imperative to enter this and only this plane and not to dissect through these structures.** The vessels can be easily identified by feeling the carotid artery pulsation and with caution developing the tissue planes. Use your fingers to feel the carotid pulsation.

Caution: It is clearly wrong to enter a plane between the oesophagus and trachea, so at all times keep the oesophagus and trachea medially and the carotid laterally. This is done by using large size Langenback retractors which are held by two assistants: one gently pulling laterally and one gently pulling medially.

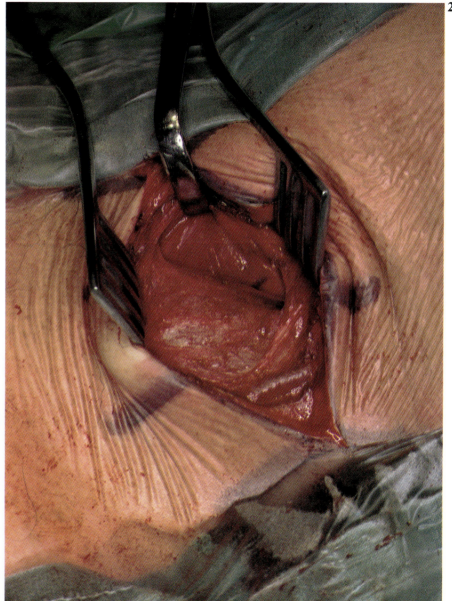

26 This plane is then further developed, to expose the cervical column.

Caution: At all times ensure your assistants do not tear the structures they are retracting. It may be necessary to ligate the medial thyroid vein during this procedure.

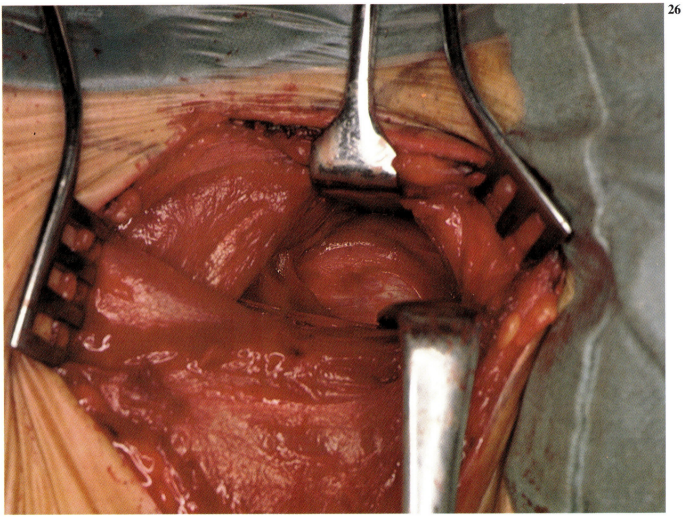

27 This plane is developed deeper, by soft tissue dissections using dental swabs, in order to expose the cervical column. The cervical column lies deep to these structures and can be palpated easily during this exposure. It is a hard structure which does not pulsate. There should be very little bleeding during this dissection, which is through easily defined planes. Use the dental swabs or the tip of your finger to gently define the planes.

Caution: At all times be gentle during this exposure and do not enter the oesophagus.

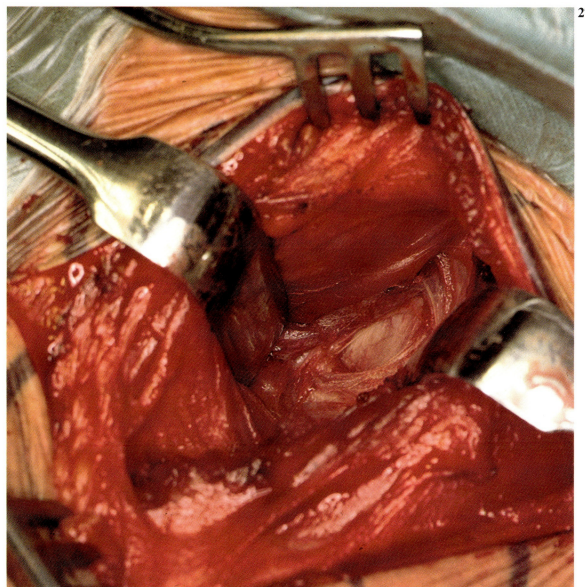

28 After the cervical column has been exposed, a needle is inserted into a disc space to identify correctly the appropriate level. An epidural needle is ideal but any needle which is long enough is suitable. This needle is used as a marker to identify the level of the cervical spine which is exposed and which will be operated upon. **It is very easy to approach the wrong cervical disc space and this step must be observed.**

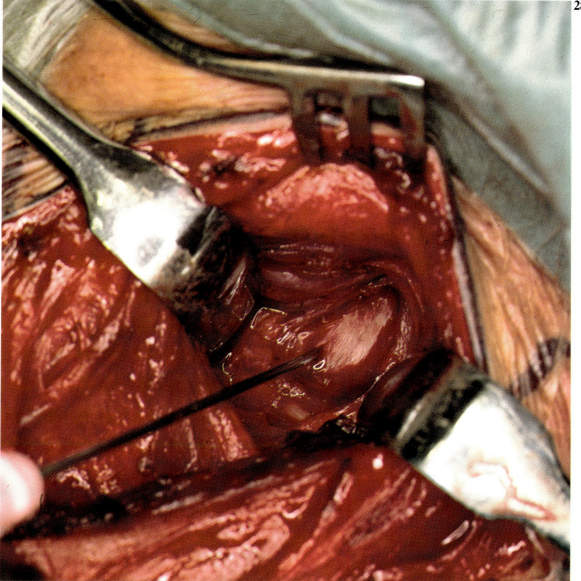

29 Under xray control the level is thus demonstrated. The xray plate is held next to the patient's neck and a lateral xray is taken.

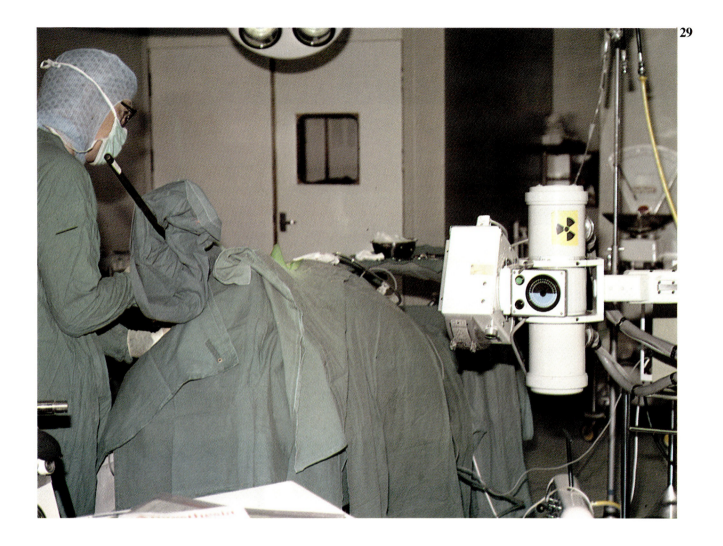

30 A lateral radiograph showing the marker in C6–7 disc space. Now it is clear which level of the cervical spine has been exposed.

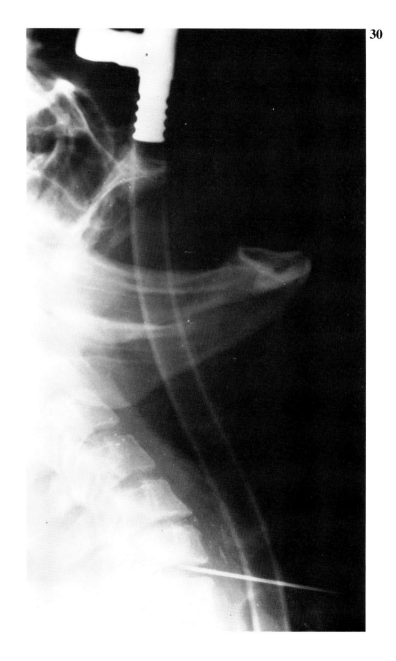

Instruments for curetting

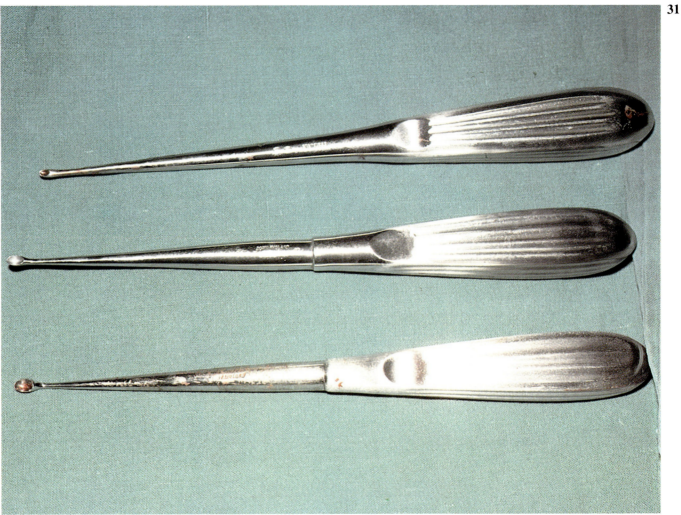

31 The disc space is then incised and curetted using a series of small curettes. Small bone nibblers can also be used to evacuate this space and disc material is removed.

Caution: Exercise great care so as not to penetrate the posterior longitudinal ligament during this manoeuvre, because immediately deep to the posterior longitudinal ligament is the spinal cord.

The lateral recesses also need curetting to remove degenerate disc material.

32 The instruments commonly used to curette out the disc.

A Pituitary rongeurs

B Small bone nibblers

C The curettes

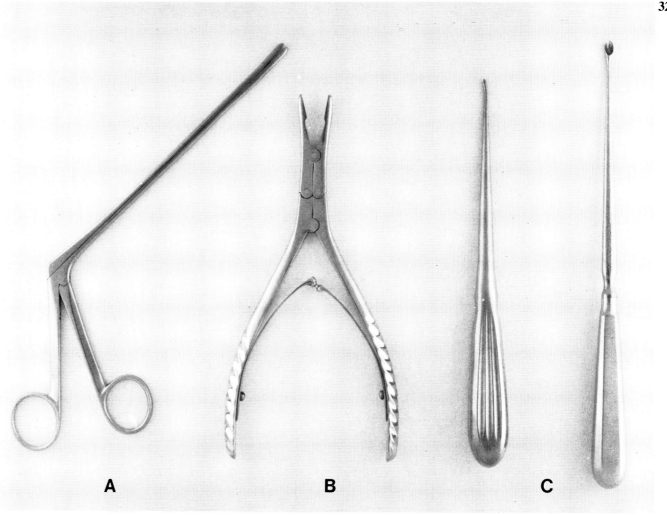

Disc removal

33 Having identified the level concerned, the anterior longitudinal ligament is incised with a long handled knife and 15 blade and the disc space exposed. The hole produced on removing the disc is expanded further and the area is developed deeper and wider, so that a reasonable area is available for the bone graft, and to remove degenerate disc material. During this time the assistants maintain steady lateral traction, keeping the soft tissues away from the operation site and also keeping the wound dry with suction.

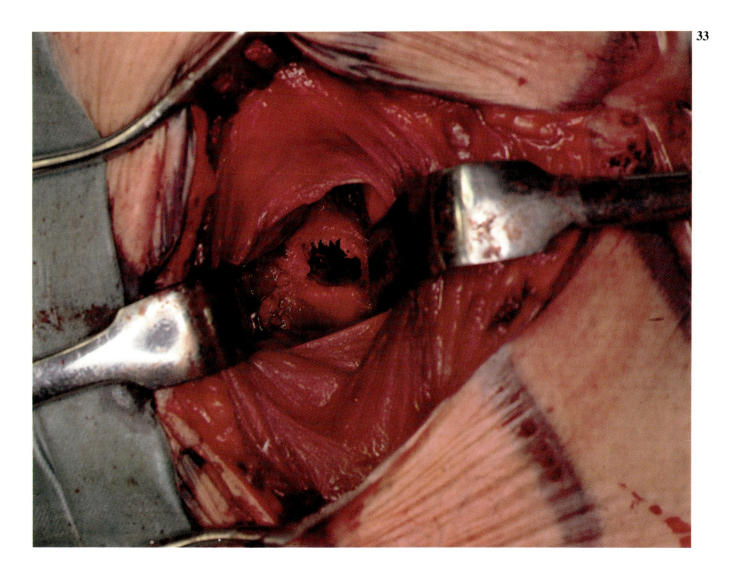

34 This illustration demonstrates the depth of the disc removed.

Caution: The posterior lip of the cervical vertebra is not removed so that the spinal cord is not exposed. This is an important part of this operation. Do not remove the posterior lip and there is also no need to expose the dura. The whole technique of this procedure remains within the disc space.

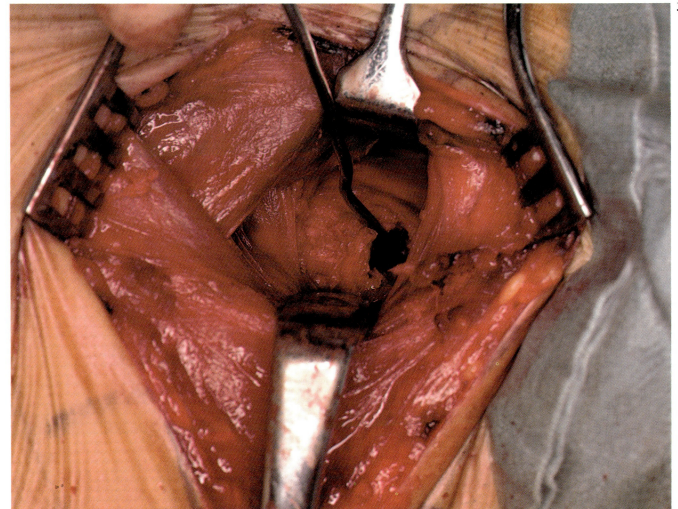

35 The quantity of disc material removed, amounts to about 2g in this patient.

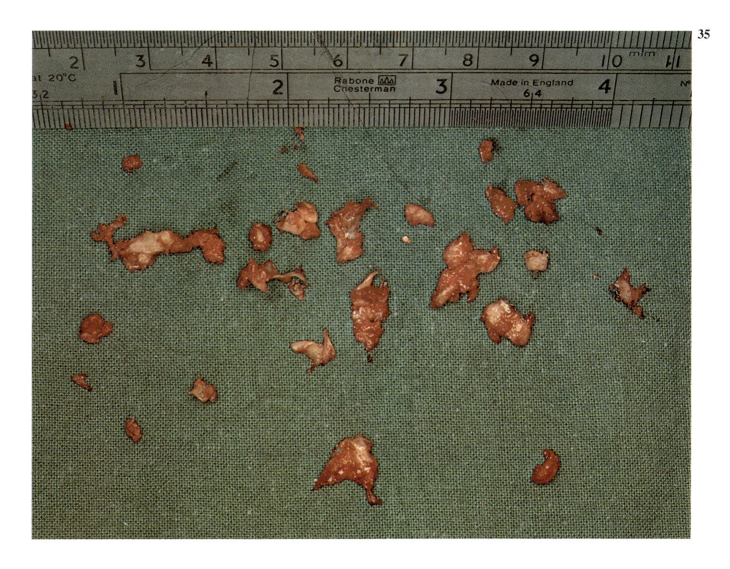

36 An H & E section of the disc material which has been removed. It is necrotic degenerate material.

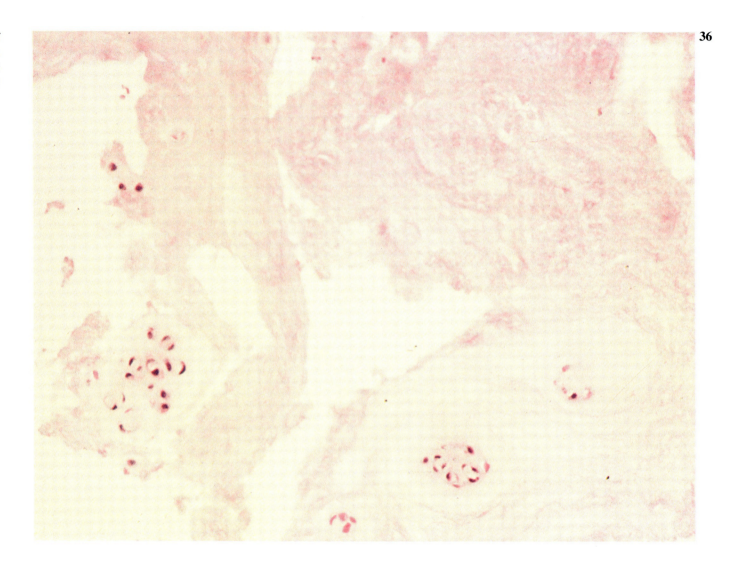

37 The end plates of the vertebrae are then undercut using a curved osteotome and a small Toffey hammer. Great care being taken not to breach the posterior lip and damage the cord. The ¼″ osteotome is bent at the tip in order to undercut the end plates and remove the cartilaginous plate, enabling the graft bed to be prepared.

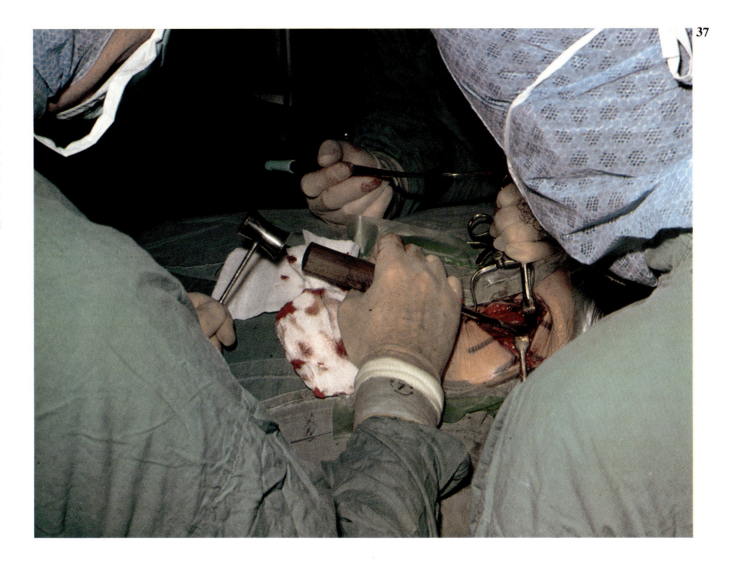

38 Retractors can be inserted to evacuate all the disc material and undercut the surface. They are specially curved and angulated so that they can then be inserted in between the cervical vertebrae.

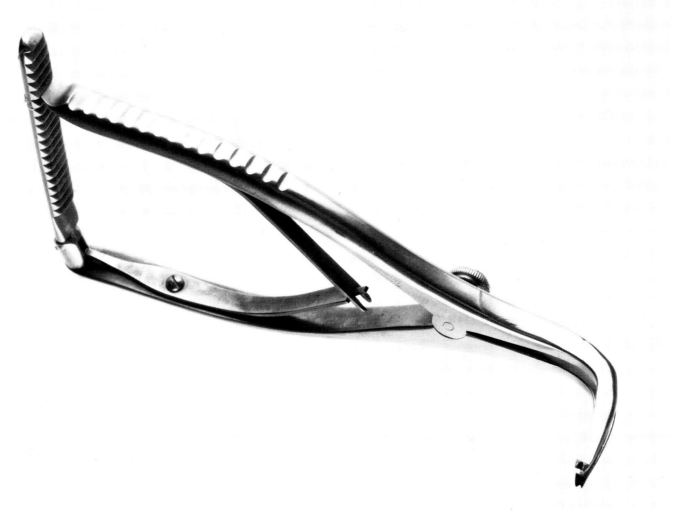

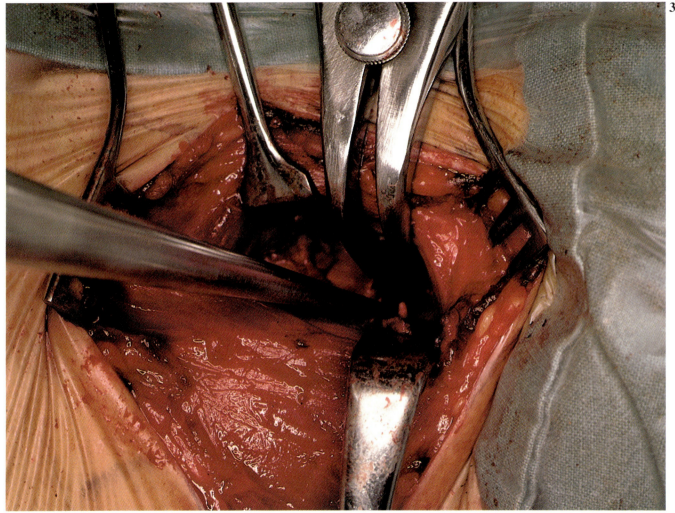

39 The retractors have been placed into the disc space, allowing the curette to remove disc material which lies in the lateral recesses.

Iliac crest exposed for graft

40 The iliac crest is then exposed for the bone graft. In this patient the left iliac crest has been exposed and the wing of the ilium will be demonstrated. Using 1″ osteotomes, blocks of iliac crest bone are cut for the bone graft.

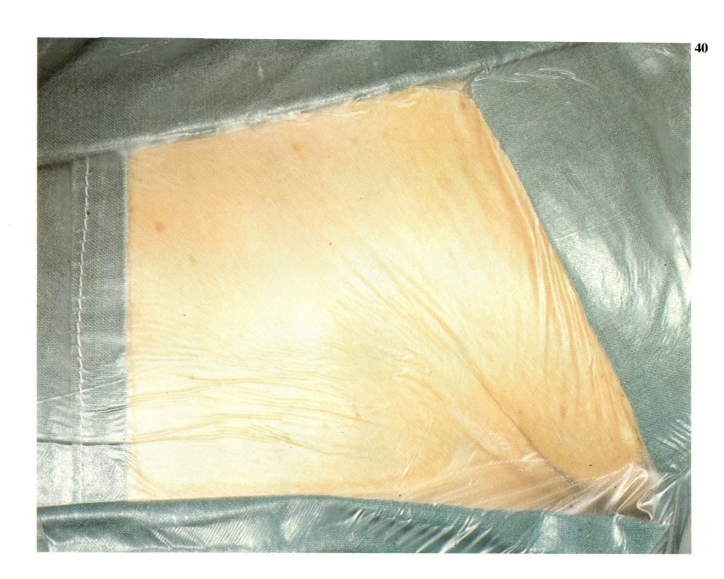

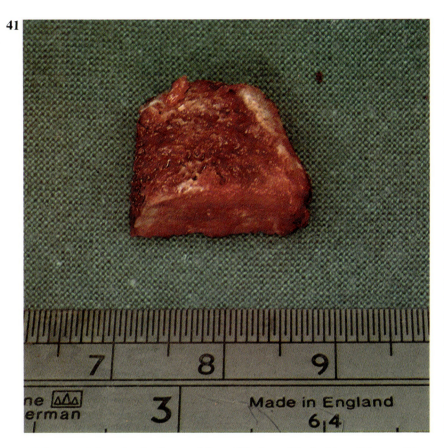

41 Bone is taken in the form of bone block and is fashioned to produce the required depth, width and height of the recipient site. This can be done with bone nibblers and bone cutters on a hard surface away from the operation site.

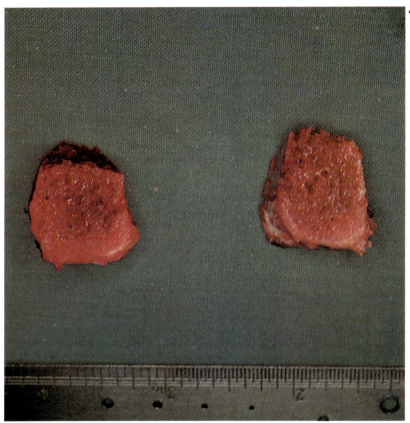

42 The graft can be cut into two separate grafts using an osteotome, if two levels of fusion are being produced.

43 With templates, the depth, width and height of the bed for the graft can be defined and then the graft can be fashioned accordingly. Using bone nibblers and cutters the graft is wedge shaped, being wide in front and tapering at its leading edge. The front cortical piece sits under the cortical bone of the exposed vertebral edge.

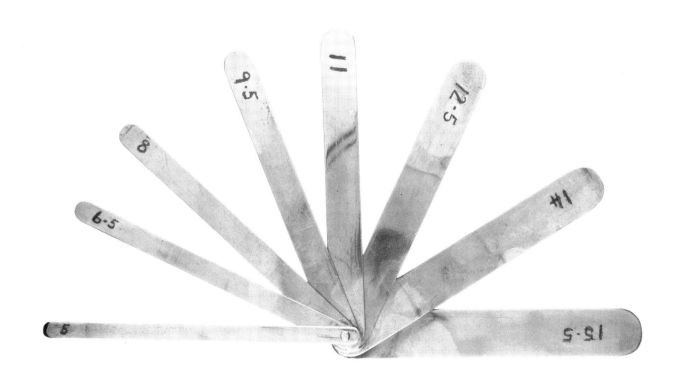

44 The bone graft is then inserted into the prepared bed in the cervical spine; the graft can be held with heavy duty toothed forceps, and the narrow edge is inserted first to sit in the disc space.

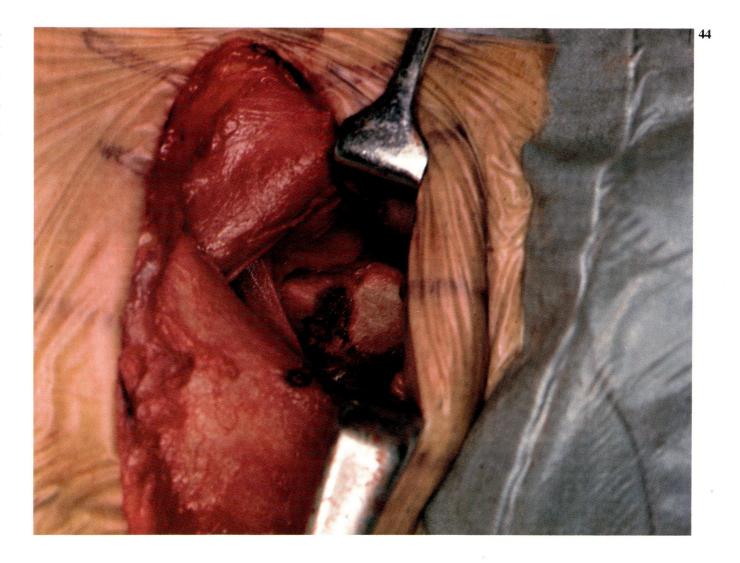

Inserting the graft

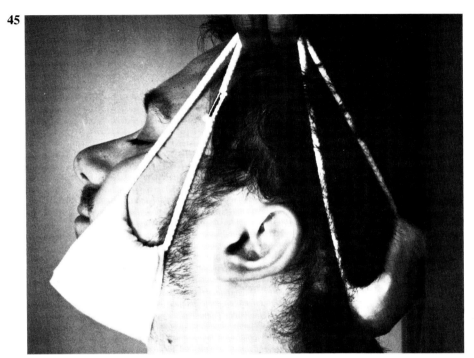

45 During this procedure the anaesthetist simultaneously applies longitudinal traction, by means of the cervical halter, which is under the drapes and placed around the chin. This steady pull provides a small degree of distraction, and is usually just enough to allow the graft to enter.

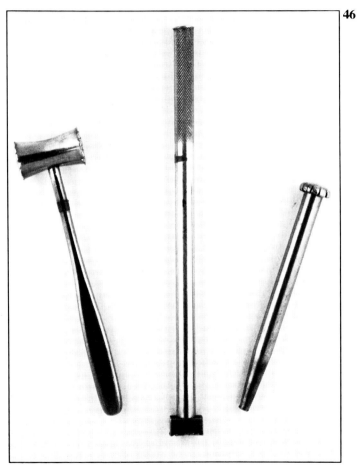

46 The graft is then driven home using a punch which can be of either size shown in this illustration, and a Toffey hammer. A few sharp short taps are all that are usually required.

47 The graft is now countersunk and sits under the overhanging surfaces of the vertebrae above and below.

Caution: Obviously DO NOT go on tapping with the punch if the graft won't enter or proceed, or you will break the graft, the overhanging bone, or worse the posterior lip and indent the cord. If the graft simply won't go, then remove it and check its dimensions with the template.

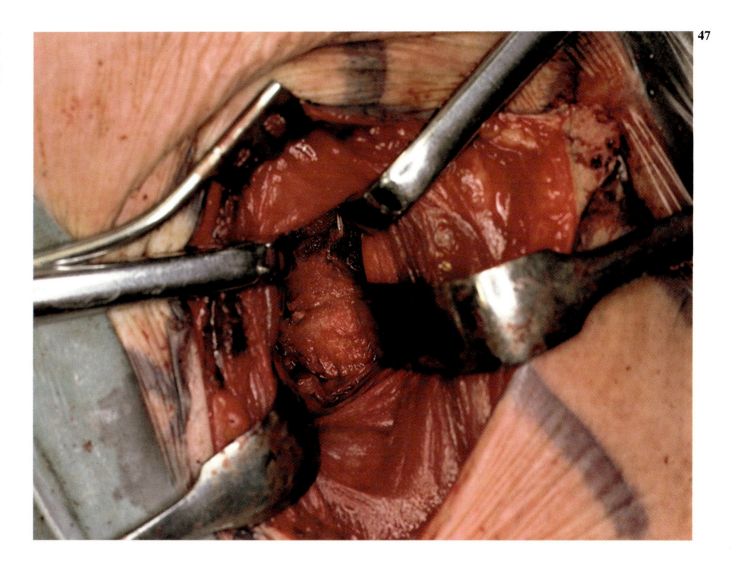

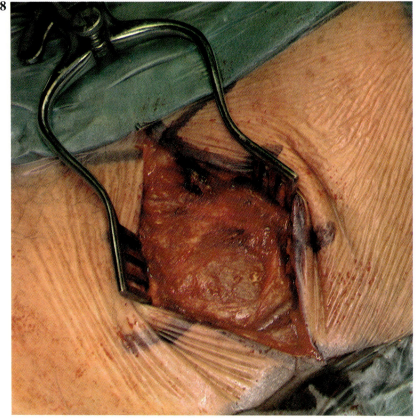

48 The neck is moved in flexion and extension by the anaesthetist to check that the graft will not fall out. If it does, use another piece of bone, because it is too small.

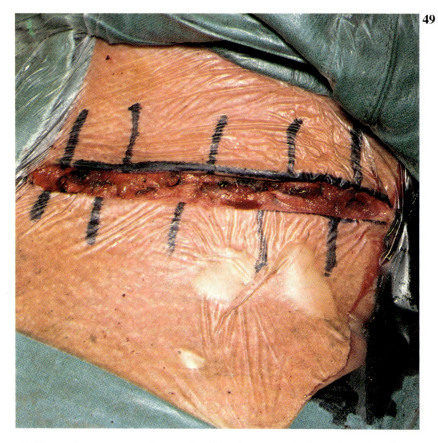

49 No drainage system is required in the neck. Unless there has been excessive bleeding during the operation. The platysma is closed with a continuous suture.

Caution: It is sensible to insert a drain into the donor site area, to prevent a haematoma forming.

Sutures and dressings

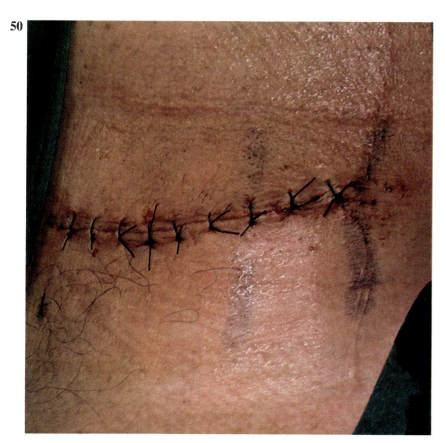

50 The skin is sutured with interrupted sutures.

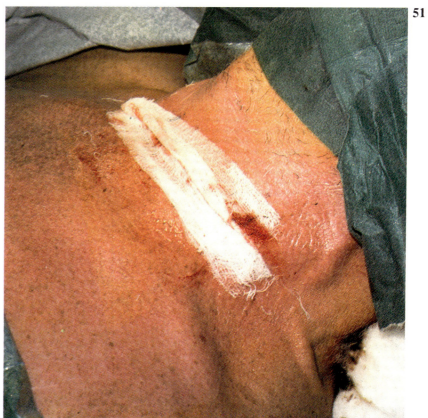

51 Dressings are applied and postoperatively the patient is nursed in bed for 24 hours and then mobilised in a soft collar, which is kept on for three weeks.

52 The postoperative check xray showing the graft in place. This may be repeated within the first week to check that the graft has not displaced.

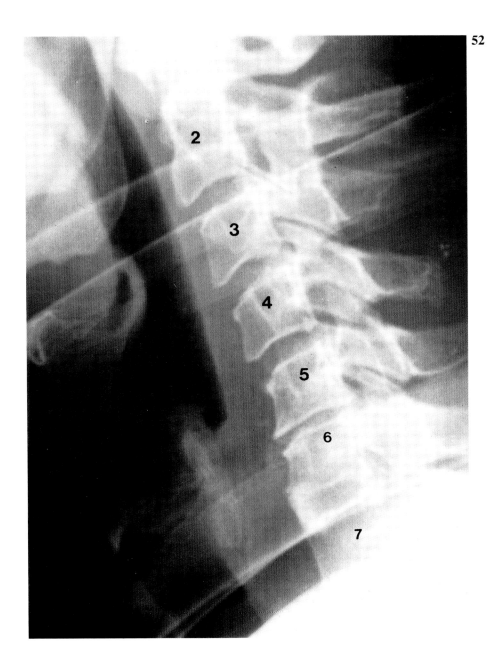

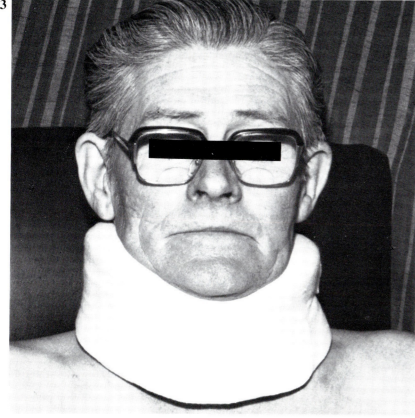
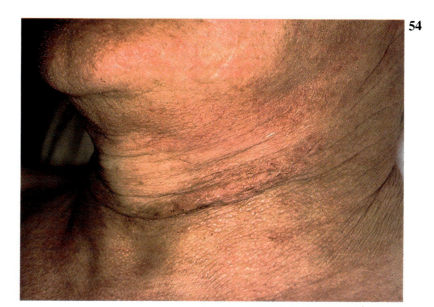
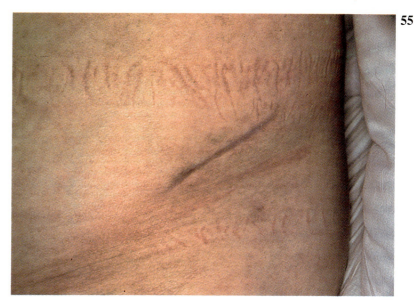

53 The patient is placed postoperatively in a cervical collar, which is made of soft material and stops the patient flexing his neck.

54 The sutures are removed at the 5th day.

55 The iliac crest sutures are removed at two weeks.

Postoperative observations

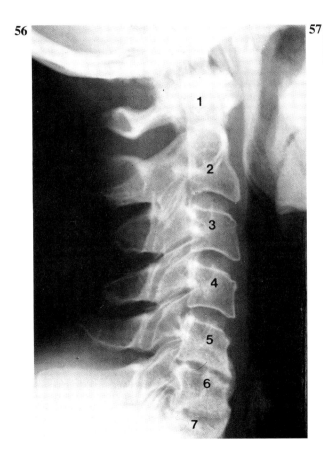
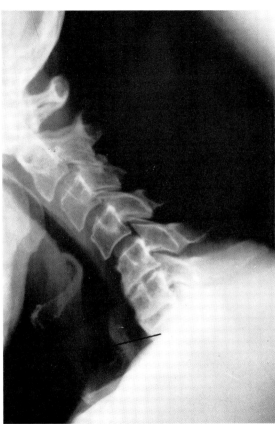
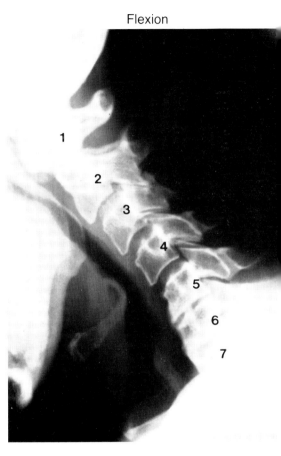

56 The postoperative xray nine months after the operation showing the bone graft has incorporated.

57 An xray of the patient 18 months later showing that a solid fusion has occurred at this level. Usually the C5–6 and C6–7 levels are the ones requiring fusion, although clearly other levels may be approached.

58 Sometimes after a two level fusion a degree instability may occur particularly at the lev above.

Extension

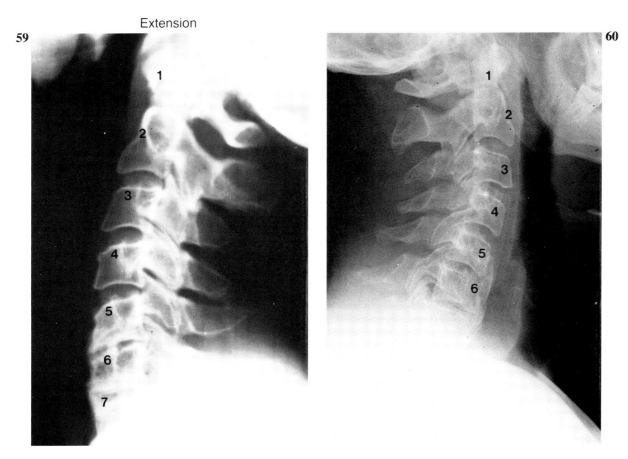

59 In this radiograph the C4–5 level appears to open and close.

60 Indeed a frank pseudoarthrosis may develop, this is more apparent when two levels have been fused.

Flexion

Extension

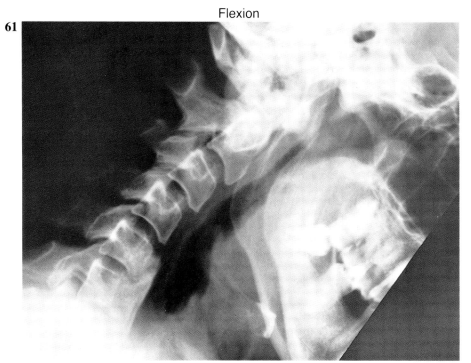
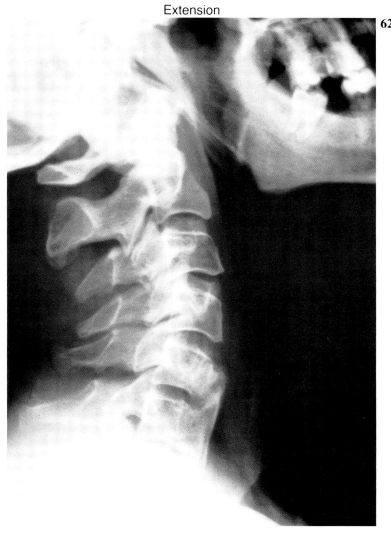

61 and 62 However, one year later the pseudoarthrosis went on to union, without surgical intervention and this is shown on flexion extension views.

63 Tumour. This approach to the spine can also be used for destruction of the cervical vertebrae, which in this patient was caused by metastatic disease from a cancer of the breast. The metastasis was exposed, curetted and a bone graft inserted.

64 One year after removal of the metastases the bone graft has solidly incorporated.

65 Trauma. This anterior approach can also be used for patients with grossly unstable cervical spine. In this patient a posterior decompression had been performed resulting in gross instability of C5 on C6.

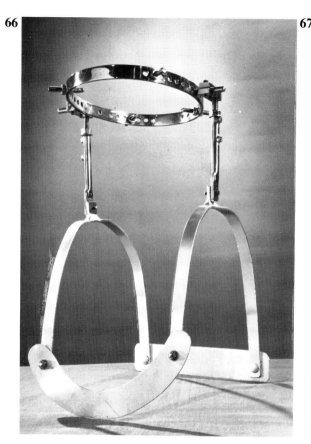
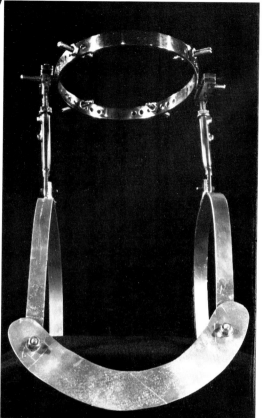
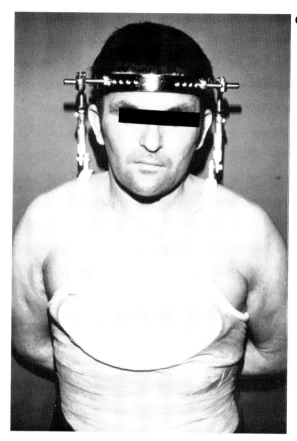

66 and 67 Before undertaking an anterior fusion, the patient was placed in a halo body fixation system, an example of which is the Princess Margaret Rose Orthopaedic Hospital Halo-Body Fixation System. This consists of a halo with four horns which is attached by self-tapping pins. The halo is linked to the body by means of vertical rods which allow for distraction, compression and rotation.

68 The patient up and about in the Princess Margaret Rose Orthopaedic Hospital Halo-Body Fixation System.

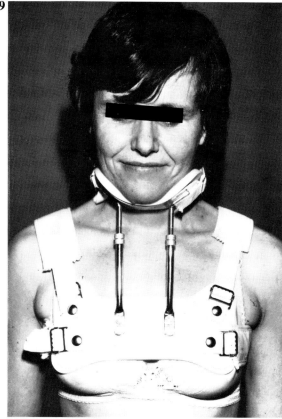

69 After six to eight weeks the patient can be placed in a four poster collar to hold the cervical spine.

Conclusion

Anterior cervical fusion can be used for 1) Cervical spondylosis in which patients undergo discectomy and fusion of the appropriate level in carefully selected patients; 2) Cervical instability following trauma producing a clear approach to the cervical spine; 3) Resecting tumours or infection involving vertebral bodies.

This approach to the cervical spine is relatively straightforward, but can produce complications.

These are:

1 Perforation of oesophagus or trachea during the dissection;
2 Damage to the common carotid artery or jugular vein during the approach to the spine;
3 Damage to the dura by broaching the posterior longitudinal ligament during the process of curetting out the degenerate disc;
4 Fracturing the vertebral bodies by over removal of bone or injudicious insertion of the retractors;
5 Damage to the nerves or cord on inserting the graft.

Bearing these problems in mind, this operation is an effective method for treating disorders of the cervical spine and is a relatively straightforward approach, provided that the planes are adhered to and excessive force is not applied.

References

1 Smith, G.W. and Robinson, R.A. 'The treatment of certain cervical spine disorders by anterior removal of the intervertebral disc and interbody fusion.' *J. Bone and Joint Surg.* **40–A,** 607–624, 1958.

2 Hughes, S.P.F., Cairns, T., Iyer, V., Liston, J., and Thomson, R.G.N., 'Halo body device.' *Paraplegia,* **22,** 260–266, 1984.

Index

References are to page numbers

Anterior longitudinal ligament incision, 39
Approach to cervical spine, 29–49
– dental swabs, use of, 33
– division of platysma, 30
– exposure of cervical column, 34
– medial thyroid vein ligation, 32
– needle insertion into disc space, 34
– palpation of cervical column, 33
– plane between trachea and oesophagus, 31–33
– radiographic confirmation of level, 35–36
Assistants, necessity for two, 20

Bone graft, 46–51
– insertion into bed, 49–50
– measurement of bed, 48
– neck movement by anaesthetist, 52
– removal, 46–47
Bone nibbler, 38
Breast metastases, 59

Cervical collar, 53, 55
Cervical disc removal, 39–42
– depth of disc removed, 40
– H & E section of disc material removed, 42
– needle insertion into, 34
– – radiographic confirmation, 35–36
– quantity removed, 41
Cervical instability, 56, 61
Cervical spondylosis, 5, 7, 62
Cervical vertebrae, 21
– posterior lip not removed, 40, 43
Clinical assessment and investigation, 7–14
– barium swallow, 12
– CAT scan, 12
– radiography, 8–10
– – contrast, 11, 14
Complications of operation, 61
Compression of cord
– CAT scan, 13
– myelogram, 13
Curettes, 37–38
Curetting of disc space, 37

Dental swabs, use of, 33
Drain
– donor site area, 52
– unnecessary in neck, 52
Dressings, 53

Fracture dislocations of cervical spine, 5

Halo-Body Fixation System, the Princess Margaret Rose Orthopaedic Hospital, 60–61

Iliac crest, exposure and removal of graft, 45–48
Infection of cervical spine, 5, 62

Medial thyroid vein ligation, 32

Neck
– deep dissection, 26–27
– superficial dissection, 23
Needle insertion into disc space, 34
Nerve root compression, assessment by contrast radiography, 11

Osteophyte formation, barium swallow demonstrated, 12
Osteotome, curved, use of, 43

Pituitary rongeur, 38
Platysma
– division, 30
– suture, 52
Posterior longitudinal ligament, 37
Postoperative care, 53–54
Preparation for surgery, 15–28
– draping, 19
– exposure of iliac crest, 19
– halter, 16
– intubation, 17, 18
– positioning, 17–18
– stability achievement, 17–18
Princess Margaret Rose Orthopaedic Hospital Halo-Body Fixation System, 60–61
Pseudoarthrosis, 57–58
Punch, 50

Retractors, 44–45

Sagittal section, lower part of head and neck, 28
Sutures in iliac crest, removal, 55
Sutures in neck, 53
– removal, 55

Templates, 48
Toffey apple, 43, 50–51
Trauma to cervical spine, 59
Tumours
– breast metastases, 59
– cervical spine, 5, 61

Xray
– clinical investigation, 8–10
– confirmation of level, 35–36
– postoperative, 54, 56
– – fusion, 56
– – pseudoarthrosis, 57–58
– two level fusion: instability at upper level, 50